teach me about
illness

Written by Joy Berry
Illustrated by Bartholomew

Published by
Peter Pan Industries
Newark, NJ 07105

Publisher: Peter Pan Industries, Newark, NJ 07105
Producer: Marilyn Berry
Editor: Orly Kelly
Consultant: Kathy McBride
Design and production: Abigail Johnston
Art Direction: Rob Lavery
Graphic coordination: Filip Associates, Inc.

I like myself.

I do not want to get sick.

I want to stay well.

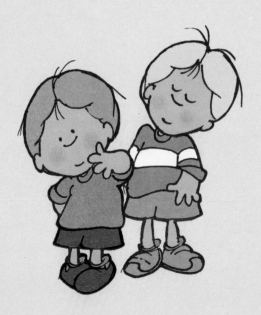

I eat good food.

It is good for me.

Good food helps me stay well.

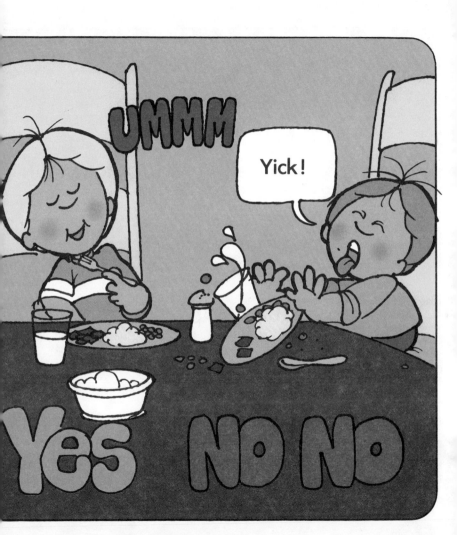

I get sick when I get too cold.

I wear warm clothes

when it is cold.

Warm clothes help me stay well.

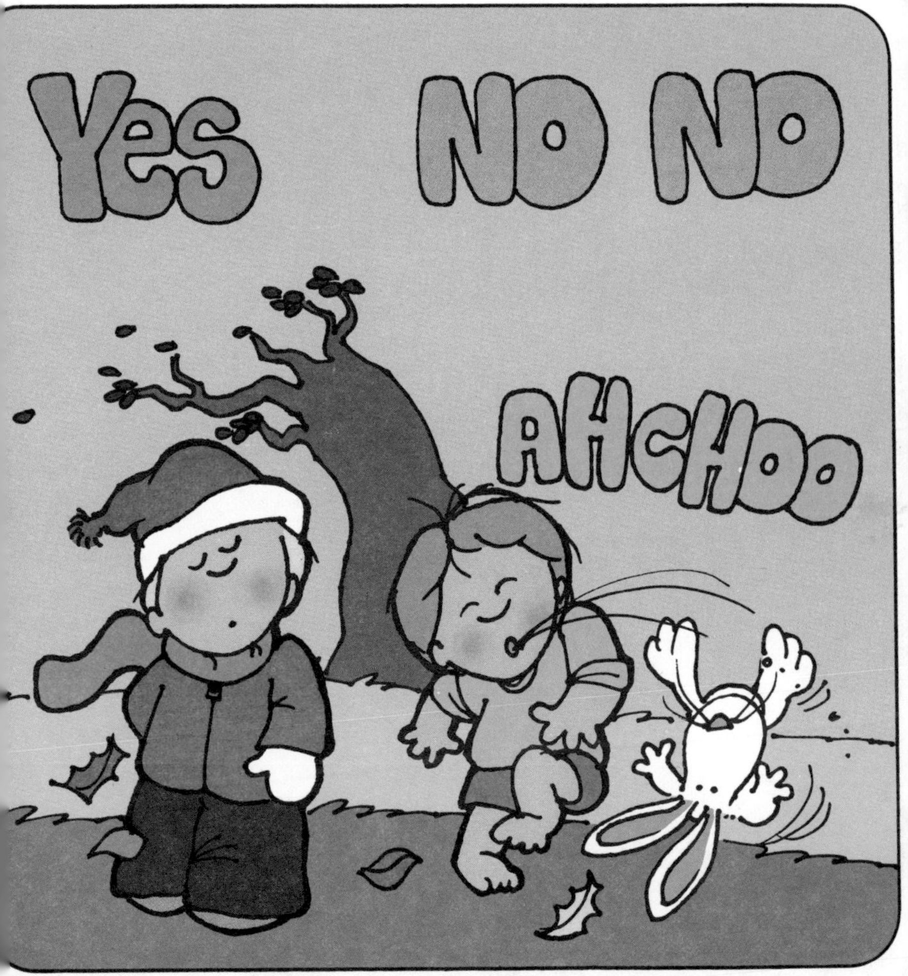
Yes
NO NO
AHCHOO

I play outside whenever I can.

It is good for me.

Fresh air and sunshine

help me stay well.

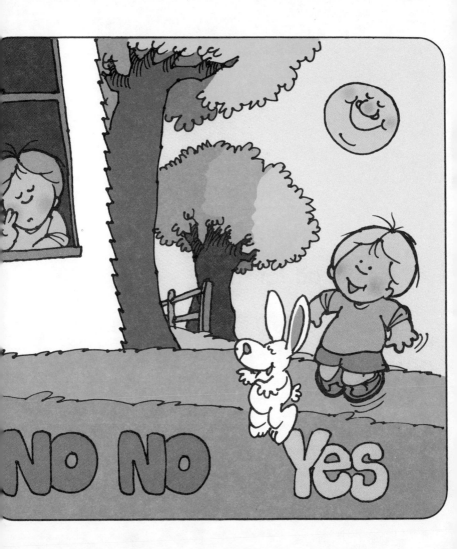

I exercise my body.

It is good for me.

Exercise helps me stay well.

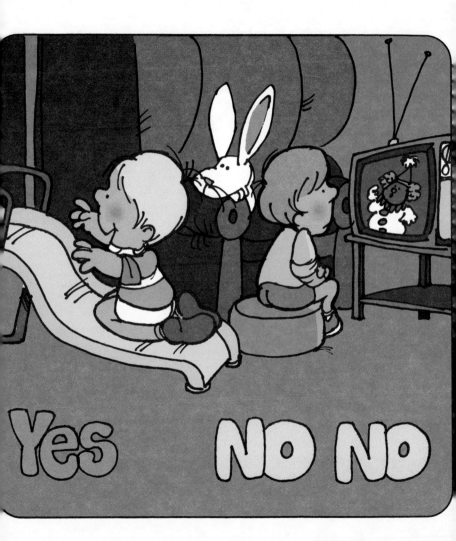

I get sick when I get too tired.

I rest when I am tired.

Rest helps me stay well.

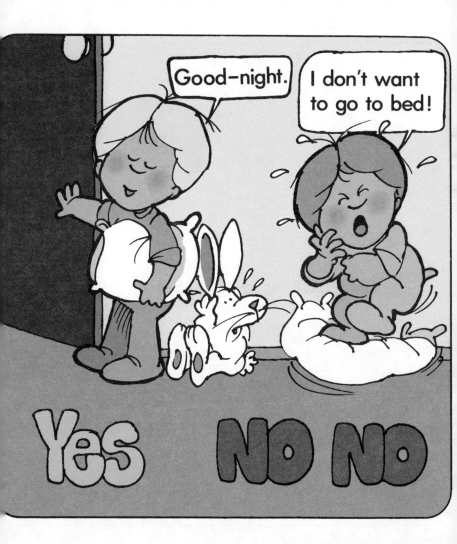

I go to the doctor's office

for check-ups.

Sometimes I get a shot.

The shot keeps me from

getting sick.

Shots help me stay well.

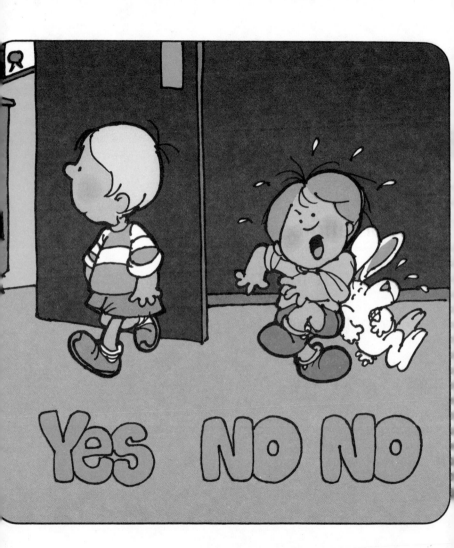

Sometimes I get sick.

I do not like being sick.

I do things to get well.

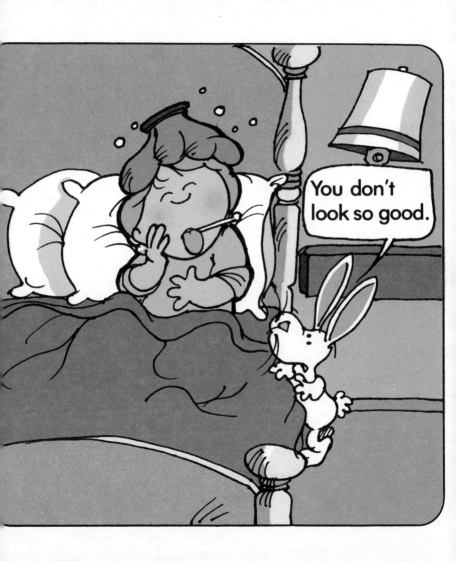

Sometimes I go to the doctor

when I am sick.

I find out what is wrong with me.

The doctor tells me

what to do to get well.

Sometimes I get a shot.

The shot helps me to get well.

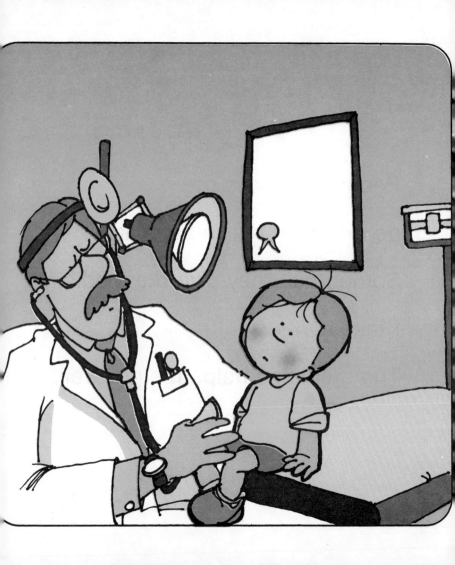

People who love me

do not want me to be sick.

Sometimes they give me medicine.

I take it.

The medicine helps me get well.

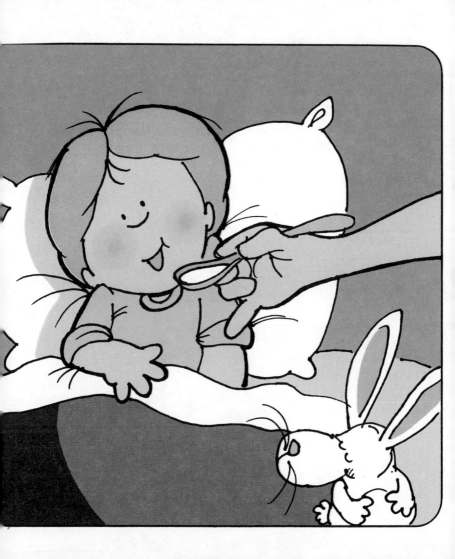

I drink lots of water and juice
when I am sick.
The water and juice
help me to get well.

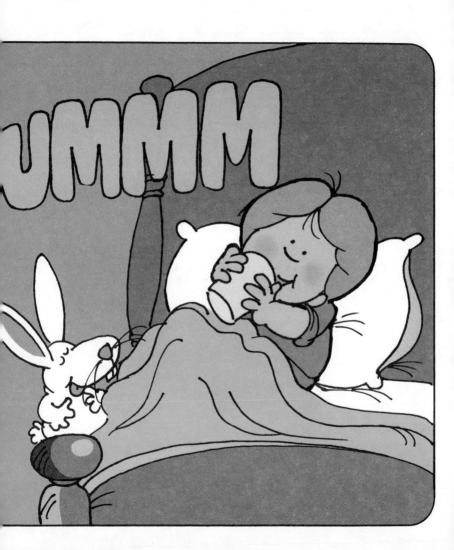

I rest when I am sick.

Resting helps me to get well.

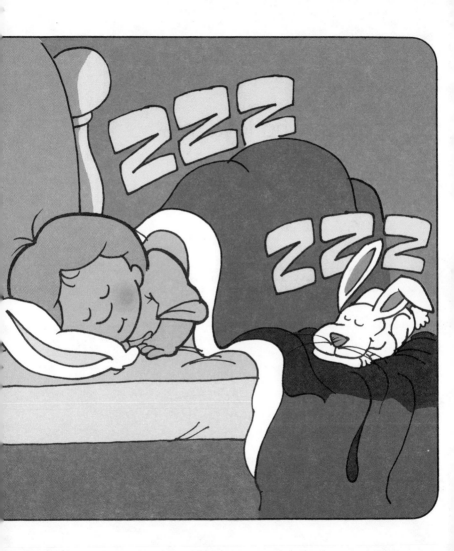

Sometimes I get hurt.

People who love me

help fix the hurt.

They clean it.

They put medicine on it.

Sometimes they put

a bandage on it.

I am careful with the hurt.

I want it to get well.

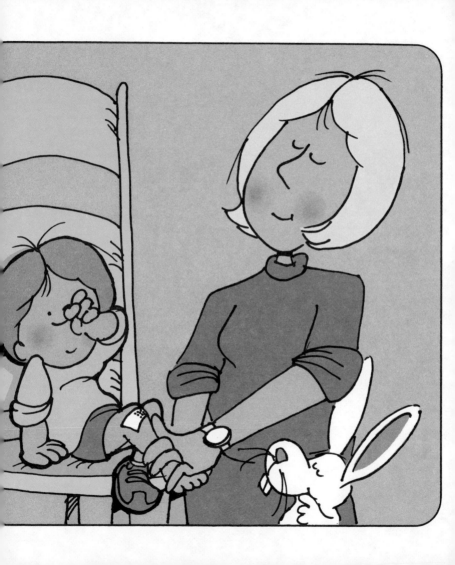

I like myself.

I want to stay well.

I take care of myself

so that I won't get sick.

I like being healthy.

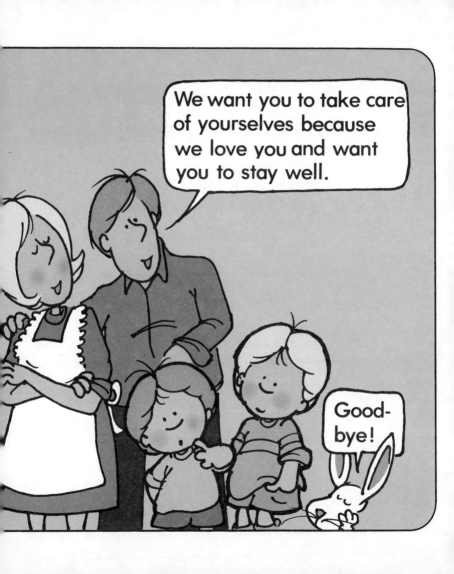

helpful hints for parents about

illness

Dear Parents:

The Purpose of this book is—

to show children what they can do to avoid illness, and
to teach sick children what they can do to help themselves
get well.

You can best implement the purpose of this book by—

Reading it to your child, and
Reading the following *Helpful Hints* and using them
whenever applicable.

AVOIDING ILLNESS

Find a caring, competent physician. Take your child to him/her for regular checkups.

Check with your doctor concerning the following recommended tests and immunizations:

2 months)	
4 months)	D.P.T. shots (pertussis, tetanus, and
6 months)	oral polio)
1 year	Tuberculin test
15 months	Measles, mumps, and rubella shots
18 months	D.P.T. plus polio booster
5 years	D.P.T. plus polio booster
10 years	D.P.T. plus polio booster

Give your child the recommended doses of vitamins and minerals every day. Be sure to include Vitamin C.

PREPARING FOR ILLNESS

Be ready to deal with any childhood illness by doing the following:

Emergency Numbers

Post these emergency numbers on or near your telephone:

- the doctor
- the fire station
- the police station
- the ambulance and/or paramedics
- the hospital
- the poison control center

Be sure you have these medicines, salves, and ointments on hand. Consult your physician for specific brand names, and read the directions carefully before administering them.

Medicines

- baby aspirin or an aspirin substitute (for fever and pain)
- a decongestant (for congestion)
- cough syrup (for coughs)
- glycerine suppositories (for constipation)
- syrup of ipecac (to induce vomiting)
- vitamin C for colds

Salves and ointments
- aloe vera (for burns)
- antibiotic salve (for cuts and scrapes)
- Vitamin E oil (to minimize scarring)
- anti-itch cream (for rashes and bites)
- hydrogen peroxide (for cleaning affected areas)
- alcohol (for sterilizing affected areas)
- sunscreen
- insect repellent
- diaper rash ointment

Miscellaneous Medical Supplies
Be sure you have these medical supplies on hand:
- a thermometer
- a humidifier
- cold compresses
- tweezers
- gauze
- an assortment of bandages

HANDLING COMMON HEALTH PROBLEMS
Here are some suggested procedures for dealing with common health problems.

Colds
- Give your child Vitamin C (consult your physician for exact dosage).
- Elevate your child's head by raising the top end of the bed or mattress.
- Increase the humidity in the bedroom with a cold-mist humidifier.

Constipation
- Have your child drink fruit juice as it is a natural laxative.
- Use a glycerine suppository when all else fails. Consult your physician first.

Cuts
- Apply pressure to stop the bleeding of a cut.
- Clean the cut with hydrogen peroxide.
- Apply Vitamin E oil.
- Bandage the cut if necessary.

Dehydration
- Put your child into a tub of running water and make a game of drinking from your hands or the faucet.
- Give your child diluted fruit juice, flavored drinks, crushed ice, or Popsicles.

Diaper Rash
- Add one-half cup baking soda to the wash cycle and one cup white distilled vinegar to the final rinse cycle when washing diapers.
- Change the diapers often.
- Wash the affected area with mild soap and clean water (avoid using prepacked wipes). If the skin is very red, splash it with warm water.
- Dry the skin with a nonasbestos hair dryer. Put the dryer on the coolest setting. Test the warmth of your own skin and hold the dryer at least six inches from the baby's skin.
- Apply moisture-repellent ointment with Vitamin A and D added.
- Discontinue giving fruit juice. (The acidity in the fruit juice may be causing the rash.)
- Offer water between meals to dilute the urine.
- Let your child go diaperless whenever possible. (The fresh air can help heal the rash.)

Heat Rash
- Apply cornstarch to the affected areas.
- Dress your child in fewer clothes.
- Put your child in cooler surroundings.

Insect Bites
- Clean the bitten area with vinegar.
- Apply a baking soda and water paste, calamine lotion, or an anti-itch cream.

Splinters
- Locate a hidden splinter by dabbing iodine on the general area. (The splinter will darken and will be easier to find.)
- Soak the affected area in warm water and/or vegetable oil.
- Numb the area with an ice cube.
- Remove the splinter with tweezers.

Sunburn
- Avoid sunburns by keeping your child in the shade, using a sunscreen lotion, and dressing him/her in a brimmed hat and high-necked shirt.
- Consult your physician if your child has a severe sunburn.
- Bathe a mild sunburn in vinegar, or give your child a tepid bath.
- Apply aloe vera to the affected area.
- Dress your child in loosely fitting clothes.
- Give your child baby aspirin if the pain persists.

Teething
- Give your child a teether to chew on. Here are some suggestions: hard breadsticks, bagels, biscuits, hard rubber "puppy rings," frozen bananas, and Popsicles.

Temperatures
A normal temperature is 99.6 degrees (rectal reading), 98.6 degrees (oral reading), and 97.6 degrees (underarm reading).
Do the following if your child's temperature is high:
- Bathe your child in tepid (not cold) water. This can be done by immersing your child in the tub or sponge-bathing him/her with a cool washcloth.
- Remove heavy clothes or blankets.
- Give your child baby aspirin (or an aspirin substitute).
- Call your physician if the high temperature persists.

The Umbilical Cord
- Keep diapers below the umbilical cord so the cord will neither be rubbed nor get wet.
- Sponge-bathe your baby until the umbilical cord falls off.

ADMINISTERING AID
Have a doll on hand when you change a bandage or treat an Injury.
Encourage your child to give the doll the same treatment he/she is receiving.
This will occupy your child and make it easier for you to administer aid.

Medicines
- Do not take medicine in front of your child. This is so his/her normal response of imitating you will not result in taking medicine without supervision.